HOW TO LOOSE WEIGHT AND LIVE A HEALTY LIFE

BY

Hannah G.M.

DEDICATION

I dedicate this book to God Almighty.

All rights reserved. No part of this publication should be reprinted or transmitted through electronic or mechanical means without prior permission by the Author, except for citations for critical cases.

Copyright Hannah G.M, 2022

TABLE OF CONTENT

CHAPTER ONE

INTRODUCTION

In the context of medicine, health, or physical fitness, the term "weight loss" refers to a decrease in the total body mass. Either accidentally, as a result of malnutrition or an underlying condition, or consciously, as a result of an endeavor to ameliorate a real or perceived state of being overweight or obese, weight loss may take place.

Cachexia is the term used to describe "unexplained" weight loss that is not the result of a decrease in calorific consumption or increased physical activity. Cachexia may be a sign of a more severe underlying medical problem.

When it comes to getting rid of excess weight, several different considerations come into play.

The fundamental idea here is that the quantity of energy that we expend in our day-to-day activities and the amount of energy that is included in the food that we consume are the two primary factors that determine our body weight. If a person's weight stays the same over time, it's probable because their caloric expenditure is equivalent to their calorie consumption.

The body will retain any unused calories as fat if they are consumed in excess. For this reason, individuals who want to reduce their body mass should either cut down on the quantity of food that they consume or boost the amount of energy that they burn via various forms of physical activity.

Losing weight on purpose is often done to better one's health and increase one's level of fitness. People who are obese or overweight stand to gain great benefits from this kind of weight loss, which includes a reduction in the associated health risks and the prevention of illnesses such as hypertension and diabetes.

Patients who consciously wish to reduce weight can accomplish so with the help of lifestyle modification measures, which mostly consist of a mix of eating fewer calories and engaging in more physical activity or exercise. Utilizing different drugs is just another approach to achieving one's weight loss goals. Patients who are morbidly obese may be candidates for bariatric surgery, which reduces the size of the stomach by surgical intervention.

On the other hand, unintended weight loss is a symptom that might be caused by a variety of other medical issues. Even when the body is at rest, illness tends to raise the requirements placed on the metabolic system. On the other hand, illnesses may cause a person to lose their appetite or make it impossible for them to eat, which leads to a lower overall calorie intake.

In addition to this, issues with digestion or the absorption of nutrients might be brought on by disorders that impact the digestive system. Also, significant losses of calories and nutrients may also take place, which is more likely in individuals who have persistent vomiting or diarrhea.

It is not necessary for individuals to adhere to a particular diet plan to successfully lose weight, such as the Atkins or Slimming World diets. They should instead concentrate on consuming fewer calories and increasing the amount of movement they do to establish a negative energy balance.

It is not necessary to make adjustments to the ratios of carbohydrates, fats, and proteins in the diet to achieve significant weight reduction. Weight loss is mostly based on lowering the overall number of calories consumed.

A decrease in body weight of 5–10 percent throughout a period of 6 months is an acceptable weight loss target to achieve to start noticing health advantages.

This objective may be accomplished by the vast majority of individuals by lowering their daily calorie consumption to a level that falls within the range of 1,000–1,600 calories.

A daily caloric intake of less than 1,000 calories will not provide the body with the necessary amount of nutrients.

Because individuals consume less energy when they are at lower body weight, the pace of weight loss often slows down after six months of dieting, and body weight typically remains stable during this time. The most effective strategy for preventing oneself from regaining weight once it has been dropped is to stick to a weight management program that includes both regular physical exercise and healthy eating habits.

Prescription weight-loss drugs may be beneficial for those who have a Body Mass Index (BMI) of 30 or above but who do not suffer from any health issues that are directly connected to their obesity. People with a body mass index (BMI) of 27 or above who are suffering from obesity-related disorders can potentially benefit from using these.

A commitment to leading a healthy lifestyle, one from which there is no "holiday," is required in order to keep the weight off once it has been lost. Even though individuals should not allow themselves to feel guilty when indulging in one-of-a-kind experiences such as a celebratory meal out, a birthday party, or a joyous holiday feast, they should still make an effort to stay on the path of eating healthily and engaging in frequent physical activity.

Those who choose to do so could discover that they are unable to concentrate. Putting on weight after it has been dropped is a lot simpler than doing the opposite.

When individuals make lasting adjustments to their lifestyle, they increase their chances of successfully losing weight and keeping it off. People who are aware of how and what they eat and who participate in daily physical activity or regular exercise will be effective both in losing extra weight and keeping it off in the long term.

This is true regardless of the exact strategies that are used to assist a person in losing weight.

Regardless of the benefits that proponents of crash diets may claim they offer, these diets are not a viable long-term option. It is vital to make progressive, persistent, and positive adjustments to one's lifestyle if one wants to lose weight healthily and maintain that weight reduction over an extended period.

For individuals who are overweight but otherwise healthy, a complete weight-loss approach must include increased opportunities for physical exercise as a mandatory component.

The capacity to create and maintain an exercise routine is one of the strongest indicators of success in the long-term treatment of overweight and obesity. Other factors include dietary changes and weight loss.

The provision of exercise facilities on military bases has the potential to enhance the effectiveness of exercise and fitness programs, both of which are essential for meeting the physical preparedness demands of the armed forces in general and especially for managing weight. The intensity, length, frequency, and kind of physical exercise that a person engages in will vary for them depending on factors such as their current medical problems, the degree of activity they have engaged in in the past, their physical limits, and their personal preferences.

A referral to an additional professional examination may be warranted, particularly in the case of persons who have more than one of the mitigating situations listed above. Even if you don't end up losing weight, engaging in physical exercise will still bring about some important advantages.

CHAPTER TWO
UDERSTAND YOUR BODY

If you question different people, you'll get a different answers about what "healthy eating" entails. It would seem that every member of a person's social circle, including healthcare experts, wellness influencers, colleagues, and family members, has a viewpoint on the most nutritious way to eat.

In addition, the inconsistent and sometimes unjustified regulations and advice that are presented in web publications about nutrition may make it very difficult to make sense of the information.

If all you want to do is eat in a manner that is good for your body and doesn't stress you out, this makes it more difficult.

The reality is that maintaining a healthy diet does not need to be difficult. It is not at all impossible to provide your body with the nutrients it needs while still indulging in the foods you like eating.

After all, food is not something to be feared, tallied, measured, or monitored; rather, it is supposed to be enjoyed.

Before we go into the specifics of what it means to eat healthily, it is vital to discuss why this topic is so important.

To begin, the caloric fuel and nutritional support that your body needs to carry out its functions come from the foods that you eat. Your health might suffer if the calories you consume or one or more of the nutrients you need are missing from your diet.

Similarly, if you consume an excessive amount of calories, you may end up gaining weight. People who are obese have a greatly greater chance of developing health conditions such as diabetes type 2, obstructive sleep apnea, and diseases of the heart, liver, and kidneys.

In addition, the quality of your nutrition influences the likelihood that you will get certain diseases, your lifespan, and your mental health.

Diets that are high in ultra-processed foods have been linked to higher rates of mortality as well as an increased risk of conditions such as cancer and heart disease. On the other hand, diets that primarily consist of unprocessed foods that are rich in nutrients have been linked to increased longevity and protection against disease.

There is some evidence that diets heavy in highly processed foods may raise the likelihood of developing depressive symptoms, in particular among those who engage in less physical activity.

What's more, if your current diet is high in ultra-processed foods and beverages like fast food, soda, and sugary cereals but low in whole foods like vegetables, nuts, and fish, it's likely that you aren't eating enough of certain nutrients, which may harm your overall health. This can be attributed to the fact that you aren't getting enough whole foods.

The majority of individuals do not need to adhere to any particular diet to feel their best; nonetheless, there are some people who, for reasons related to their health, must avoid certain foods or prefer to adopt diets.

That is not to mean, however, that there aren't any beneficial eating patterns out there for you to follow.

For instance, some individuals have the greatest sense of well-being while adhering to a low-carb diet, while others thrive on diets that are abundant in carbohydrates.

To be clear, though, eating healthily has absolutely nothing to do with following any particular diet or set of dietary guidelines. A straightforward definition of "healthy eating" is making your health a top priority by supplying your body with meals rich in essential nutrients.

The particulars may vary from person to person based on factors such as their region, level of wealth, the culture and civilization they come from, their affinity for certain flavors, and so on.

If you're like the majority of people, you're probably eager to know when you can expect to start seeing results from your efforts to lose weight after you've started those efforts.

At the same time, you may also be interested in finding out whether the weight you are losing is coming from muscle or water, or whether it is coming from fat.

The steps of weight reduction are broken down and discussed in this book.

Phase 1: Sudden and significant weight reduction.
During the initial stage of weight reduction, you will likely experience the greatest amount of weight loss and will become aware of changes in both your look and the

way your clothes fit. It normally occurs somewhere between the first four and six weeks.

The majority of the weight loss that occurs during this stage comes from the body's reserves of carbohydrates, protein, and water, with some of the weight loss coming from body fat.

Individuals who follow a low carb or keto diet are more likely to experience rapid weight loss than those who follow a low-fat diet. This is because people who follow these diets tend to exhaust their body's carb reserves more quickly, along with water.

On the other hand, the evidence is still inconclusive as to whether a low-carb or keto diet gives an advantage for total weight reduction over a low-fat diet for a lengthy time.

Your pace of weight reduction may also be affected by factors other than your diets, such as your age, gender, initial weight, and amount of physical activity. These factors can all play a role.

For instance, males are more prone to have rapid weight loss than women, and older persons may experience rapid weight loss in comparison to their younger counterparts, although some of this weight loss may be due to muscle.

On the other hand, having a greater beginning weight and increasing the frequency with which you exercise both increases the likelihood that you will lose weight more quickly.

Phase 2: Loss of weight more gradually

In the second stage, weight loss happens at a considerably slower pace, but the majority of it comes from body fat. This stage typically begins after 6 weeks and continues forward.

You may hit a weight loss plateau at some point, which is a time during which you lose very little or no weight.

Plateaus in weight reduction may be caused by metabolic adaptations, which slow down your metabolism and reduce the number of calories you burn during exercise.

On the other hand, weight loss plateaus are more often experienced because many diets are excessively restrictive and difficult to adhere to, which leads individuals to divert from them.

As a result of this, it is essential to adhere to a dietary pattern that is suitable for your way of life as well as your own tastes to be able to keep it so over time.

CHAPTER THREE
KNOW THE PROCESS INVOLVED

In any scenario, you'll probably need to make changes to your food and lifestyle throughout some time to achieve your objective.

feel loose, or you may have discovered that you can wear an item that had been stashed away in the back of your closet.

Develop your competence in an endeavor that you've been putting off (such as being able to keep up with the kids without getting out of breath).

It's possible that you feel that you have more energy, that activities need less effort for you, or that you're sleeping better.

How to reduce weight in a manner that is good for your health

Maintaining a healthy weight after weight loss requires a commitment to a healthy lifestyle that lasts a lifetime. Don't try to overhaul everything at once; rather, focus on making a few manageable adjustments to your food and level of physical activity in the initial stages of your journey.

You may reduce the amount of fat on your body by making a few simple adjustments to the way you eat, including the following:

- If you want to lessen the likelihood of engaging in yo-yo dieting, you should steer clear of crash diets and other types of unsustainable eating plans.

- Make it a point to consume foods that belong to each of the five food categories recommended by the Australian Guide to Healthy Eating.

- Increase your consumption of fruit and vegetables, especially veggies, since they are often low in kilojoules and rich in fiber, both of which contribute to a feeling of fullness.

- Be conscious of the quantities of food and beverages that you put into your body since the larger the serving size, the more calories it will have.

- Cut down on meals that are heavy in added fat, saturated fat, sugar, and salt in order to improve your health.

- Make alcoholic beverages, soft drinks, candies, and snack foods an "extra" that you allow yourself sometimes.

The average adult should limit themselves to no more than one or two "treats" every day. If you are overweight or don't get enough exercise, you may want to cut down to fewer than one treat each day.

How many drinks of the typical size do you have throughout a week?

Make an effort to strike a balance between an "extra" meal and additional activity. The more calories you burn off, the more snacks you'll have room for in your diet. Keep in mind that you should only add additional foods once you have satisfied your nutritional requirements with selections from the food categories that are considered to be healthier.

- Avoid cutting out any of the dietary groups. Instead, choose your selections from a diverse array of meals each day and prioritize 'whole' foods that have been little processed.

- Maintain a consistent eating routine and don't deviate from it.

- Water should be substituted for sugary beverages.

You should try to avoid utilizing food as a source of consolation, especially when you are feeling unhappy, irritated, or worried. Investigate additional healthy coping methods for dealing with these sensations (such as going for a walk, reading a book, having a bath, or listening to music).

Consider the evidence: even if it is possible to consume an entire family-sized block of chocolate in a single sitting, you would need to jog for almost 2.5 hours or walk for over 6 hours to burn off the energy that it contains. Easy strategies to increase your level of physical activity (energy out)

Remember that engaging in physical exercise does not need to be taxing, although we may find reasons not to, such as being excessively busy or exhausted.

Even very modest levels of physical exercise, such as walking for thirty minutes a day, may assist speed up our metabolic rate and make it easier to shed excess pounds. We may also discover that we are less exhausted and have more energy to engage in the activities that bring us delight.

When you first begin, be sure to take things carefully. Simply increasing the amount that you walk about when you're awake will help you achieve your exercise goals. The human body was made to move, and there are advantages to be gained from engaging in any kind of physical exercise.

Give these easy recommendations a shot:

Engage in physical exercises of a moderate intensity throughout the day – (go for a walk, do some gardening or mowing the lawn).

Even if you have to spend the day sitting in a car, make an effort to get some exercise. Parking farther away or using public transportation are your two options.

It is preferable to have face-to-face conversations with coworkers rather than sending emails to them while you are at work.

If you spend most of your day sitting at work, consider getting a desk that allows you to stand up while working or holding meetings in a standing position.

When going shopping, park farther away from the entrance.

Participate in a sport or hobby that brings you delight.

For shorter distances, consider walking rather than driving the automobile.

Get off the subway, bus, or tram one stop early, and then walk the remaining distance to your destination.

Increase the amount of time you spend with your family and friends playing games outside.

Walk the dog every day.

Use the stairs rather than the elevators.
Pick activities you like doing rather than ones you convince yourself are healthy for you. This increases the likelihood of you remaining with them as a result.

Use your imagination and pick up a hobby that you liked doing when you were a kid.
Keep things straightforward; there's no need to go the extra mile (unless you want to). Look for little methods to raise your activity level so that you may start increasing the quantity of energy you burn, which will lead to weight loss if you do it.

CHAPTER FOUR
SET GOALS AND IMPLEMENT

In the years 2015 and 2016, the Centers for Disease Control and Prevention (CDC) estimated that there were around 93.3 million individuals in the United States who were obese. This represents 39.8 percent of the total population when expressed as a number.

The chance of developing major health issues, such as heart disease, high blood pressure, and type 2 diabetes, might be increased when an individual carries extra body weight.

Regardless of the benefits that proponents of crash diets may claim they offer, these diets are not a viable long-term option. It is vital to make progressive, persistent, and positive adjustments to one's lifestyle if one wants to lose weight healthily and maintain that weight reduction over an extended time.

Do you find it difficult to reduce your weight and then maintain the loss over time? Don't be concerned... you're not the only one that feels this way.

The good news is that we can lose weight, keep it off, and boost our health for the rest of our lives simply by making some simple changes to our eating and physical activity habits, in ways that we can sustain and maintain for the rest of our lives (rather than by dieting for a limited amount of time), in ways that we can sustain and maintain for the rest of our lives.

Setting attainable objectives is a fantastic place to start in order to get your old routines back in shape.

Keeping a simple diary for a few weeks to record our eating habits and levels of physical activity is one way to get started with this. Keeping such a diary can assist us in establishing goals that are within our reach and in organizing the positive changes we need to make in order to achieve those goals.

This book offers ten suggestions for better management of one's weight.

10 helpful hints for achieving lasting weight reduction

People are able to successfully lose weight and keep it off by following a series of actions that are within their reach. These include;

1. Consume a wide variety of meals that are rich in color and nutrients.

Eat a diversified, healthful diet.

The cornerstone of a human diet should consist of nutritious meals as well as nutritious snacks. Making ensuring that fifty percent of each meal is comprised of fruits and vegetables, twenty-five percent of whole grains, and twenty-five percent of protein is a straightforward method for developing a meal plan. The recommended daily intake of fiber is between 25 and 30 grams. a daily dose of Trusted Source (g).

Reduce your consumption of saturated fats as well as trans fats from your diet. There is a high correlation between the consumption of saturated fats and the occurrence of coronary heart disease.

The use of monounsaturated fatty acids (MUFA) and polyunsaturated fatty acids (PUFA), both of which are kinds of unsaturated fat, is an alternative option for individuals.

The following foods are good for your health and are often high in various nutrients:
new and uncooked fruits and veggies

fish\slegumes\snuts\sseeds

cereals made from entire grains, such as oatmeal, and brown rice

The following categories of food should be avoided:

meals that have had more oils, butter, and sugar added to their foods that are fatty and either red or processed meats

baked goodies

bagels

white bread

foods that are processed

When certain foods are eliminated from a person's diet, there is a possibility that the individual may experience a shortage of certain essential vitamins and minerals. A person who is trying to lose weight might benefit from the guidance of a nutritionist, dietitian, or another kind of healthcare expert on the best ways to ensure they are getting the necessary amounts of certain nutrients.

2. Keep a record of your daily food intake and weight.

When it comes to effectively reducing weight, self-monitoring is one of the most important factors. People may keep track of every item of food that they eat daily by keeping a paper diary, using a smartphone app, or visiting a specialized website. They may also assess their development by keeping a weekly weight log and comparing it to previous readings.

Those who can monitor their progress in manageable chunks and note any changes in their appearance are considerably more likely to remain committed to a plan for weight reduction.

Using a body mass index (BMI) calculator, individuals are also able to monitor their own body mass index (BMI).

3. Make physical activity and exercise a consistent part of your routine.

One may benefit from losing weight by engaging in regular physical exercise. Exercising consistently is critical for maintaining both one's physical and mental health. It is generally essential for effective weight reduction to increase the amount of time spent being physically active in a manner that is both disciplined and intentional.

An optimal amount of physical exercise for the body is one hour per day at a moderate level, such as brisk walking. If a person is unable to exercise for one hour each day, the Mayo Clinic recommends that they try to exercise for a minimum of one hundred fifty minutes each week.

People who do not often engage in physical activity should begin by exercising for a shorter duration at a lower intensity and gradually work their way up to a longer duration. This strategy is the most sustainable method to guarantee that regular exercise becomes a part of their lives, and it is one that you should consider doing.

People may find that keeping track of their physical activity yields similar psychological benefits to those documenting their meals while trying to lose weight as recording their meals. After logging their food consumed and the amount of activity they do, a person may use one of the several free smartphone applications that are available to monitor their calorie deficit.

If someone who is new to exercise finds the idea of a complete workout to be overwhelming, they may start by engaging in activities such as those listed below to raise their levels of physical activity:

use the stairway, rake leaves, walk a dog, gardening, dancing, play outdoor activities, parking farther away from a building entrance. People who have a lower chance of developing coronary heart disease are less likely to need a medical evaluation before beginning an exercise routine.

However, a preliminary medical examination could be a good idea for some individuals, such as those who have diabetes. Anyone unsure about the amounts of exercise that are considered safe should consult with a medical professional.

4. Eliminate liquid calories

It is quite feasible to eat hundreds of more calories daily just by consuming sugar-sweetened beverages such as soda, tea, juice, or alcohol. These are referred to as "empty calories" since they increase a person's overall calorie intake without providing any additional nutritious value.

A person shouldn't drink smoothies unless they're going to use them to substitute for a meal; otherwise, they should stick to water, unsweetened tea, and coffee, or black coffee. The taste of water may be enhanced by adding a few drops of fresh lemon or orange juice.

Avoid confusing dehydration with hunger. A sip of water may often sate the appetite in between regularly planned meals for a person. [Case in point:] [Case in point:]

5. Determine the appropriate serving size and maintain portion control.

Gaining weight is possible by consuming an excessive amount of any food, even veggies with fewer calories.

As a result, individuals have to steer clear of gauging the appropriate portion size for themselves or ingesting food straight from the packaging. It is best to use measuring cups and recommendations for appropriate portion sizes. When you guess, you tend to overestimate, which increases the risk that you will consume a bigger quantity than is required.

When eating out, the following size comparisons might help keep track of the amount of food consumed:

A golf ball is equal to one-fourth of a cup.

A tennis ball is equal to one-half of a cup.

One cup is equal to a baseball.

A standard handful of nuts is one ounce (oz).

1 teaspoon equals one face on a die

A thumb tip is equal to one tablespoon.

A deck of cards equals three ounces of beef.

1 sliver is equal to 1 DVD

Although they are not accurate measurements, they may assist a person in controlling the amount of food they consume when more precise equipment is not accessible.

6. Chew with awareness

The practice of mindful eating, in which one is completely aware of why, how, when, and where they eat as well as what they consume, is beneficial to a large number of individuals.

Increasing one's awareness of one's body may directly lead to improved dietary choices that are better for one's health.

People who engage in the practice of mindful eating often make an effort to eat more slowly, appreciate each bite, and focus their attention on the flavor of the food they are eating. The body can detect all of the signals for fullness if a meal is stretched out for twenty minutes.

It is vital to concentrate on feeling content rather than full after a meal, and it is also crucial to keep in mind that many foods that are marketed as "all-natural" or low-fat are not always the healthiest option.

Regarding the option that they choose for their lunch, individuals may additionally think about the following questions:

Is it a "good bargain" considering the number of calories it contains?

Will I feel satisfied after eating it?

Are the components good for your body?

If there is a label, what percentage of the daily recommended salt intake does it have?

7. Stimulus and cue control

There are a lot of social and environmental triggers that might induce needless eating. For instance, some individuals have a higher propensity to overeat while doing anything else, like watching television. Some people have problems handing a bowl of sweets to another person without helping themselves a bit first.

People who are aware of the factors that may prompt them to want empty-calorie snacks are better able to devise strategies to modify their daily routines to reduce the impact of these factors.

8. Prepare in advance

It is possible to achieve more substantial weight reduction by stocking a kitchen with foods that are conducive to dieting and developing planned meal plans.

People who want to lose weight or maintain their weight loss should rid their kitchen of processed or junk foods and make sure they have the goods on hand to prepare straightforward meals that are good for them. If you do this, you may avoid eating hastily, without a strategy, and carelessly.

Making your meal selections ahead of time, either before going to a social function or a restaurant, may also make the procedure simpler.

9. Participate in social support groups
Embracing the support of loved ones is an essential component of a weight reduction journey that is effective.
Some individuals may want to ask friends or family members to join them, while others may want to utilize social media to discuss their progress instead of inviting others to participate in the activity with them.

Other potential sources of assistance might include the following:

a supportive social network, therapy sessions on an individual basis, fitness groups or partners, and workplace help programs for employees

10. Keep a good attitude.
The process of losing weight takes place over time, and a person may experience feelings of frustration if they do not see the pounds fall off at the pace that they had expected.

When you are trying to lose weight or maintain your current weight, there may be days that are more challenging than others. A person has to be able to keep going even when the process of changing themselves appears impossible, for their weight reduction program to be effective.

Some individuals may need to reevaluate their objectives, which might include revising the overall amount of calories they want to consume or the routines in which they engage in physical activity.

The most essential thing is to retain a good mindset and be consistent while working toward the goal of conquering the obstacles that stand in the way of healthy weight reduction.

CHAPTER FIVE

WATCH YOUR DIET

There are good eating habits that are also helpful for healthy living and they are as follows:

- Consume a diet high in nutrients that are mostly composed of foods derived from plants rather than those derived from animals.
- Consume several servings of bread, whole grains, pasta, rice, and potatoes every single day.
- Consume a wide range of fresh vegetables and fruits, ideally ones that are grown in the immediate area, many times daily (at least 400g per day).

- Reduce the amount of fat you eat (it should make up no more than 30 percent of your daily calories), and try to replace the majority of the saturated fat you eat with unsaturated fat.

- Beans, legumes, lentils, fish, poultry, or lean cuts of meat should take the place of fatty cuts of meat and animal products.

- Make use of milk and other dairy products (kefir, sour milk, yogurt, and cheese) that are low in both fat and salt content.

- Choose meals that have a minimal amount of sugar, and eat free sugars in moderation while reducing the number of times you consume sugary beverages and sweets.

- Choose a low-salt diet. The recommended maximum daily consumption of salt is one teaspoon (5 grams), which includes the salt that is found in bread as well as other processed, cured, and preserved foods. (In regions where there is an iodine shortage, the iodization of salt ought to be mandatory.)

The World Health Organization does not impose any specific limitations on the amount of alcohol that may be consumed since the research suggests that the best thing for one's health is to abstain from drinking at all. Nevertheless, drinking less is preferable.

Make sure the food is prepared in a sanitary and risk-free manner. Cooking methods such as steaming, baking, boiling, or microwaving may help cut down on the quantity of added fat.

Encourage exclusive breastfeeding during the first six months of a child's life, then gradual introduction of healthy, age-appropriate meals as a supplement beginning around the sixth month mark. It is important to encourage breastfeeding to continue during the first two years of a child's life.

CHAPTER SIX

our capacity to maintain a healthy weight under stressful conditions might be substantially impacted. Additionally, it might impede your efforts to reduce your body fat. The connection between stress and weight increase is undeniable, regardless of whether it is due to elevated levels of the stress hormone cortisol, unhealthy habits that are triggered by stress, or any mix of the two.

The Connection Between Anxiety and the Hormone Cortisol

Researchers have known for a long time that increases in the stress hormone cortisol may contribute to an increase in one's overall body mass. Your adrenal glands secrete adrenaline and cortisol while you're under pressure, and as a direct consequence of this, glucose, which is your major source of energy, is released into your circulation.

This is done in order to provide you with the vitality you need to get away from a potentially dangerous scenario (also known as the fight or flight response). After the danger has passed, the rush of adrenaline you experienced will wear off, and the surge in your blood sugar will begin to fall. This is the point at which cortisol goes into high gear to immediately refill your energy reserve.

Sugar Cravings and the Hormone Cortisol

Sugar cravings are about to begin. When you're under a lot of pressure, the first thing that probably comes to mind is something sweet to eat since sugar gives your body the fast energy it believes it needs.

Consuming a large quantity of sugar results in your body developing a propensity to retain sugar, which is particularly noticeable after experiencing stressful events. The majority of this energy is stored in the form of abdominal fat, which is known for being notoriously difficult to lose. And so the vicious cycle begins: you feel stressed, and your body releases cortisol, which causes weight gain; you then want more sweets, eat more sugar, and continue to gain weight.

The Role of Cortisol in Metabolism

Cortisol can slow down your metabolism, even if you are not consuming meals that are heavy in fat and sugar, which makes it more difficult to lose weight.

In 2015, researchers from Ohio State University fed women a high-fat, high-calorie dinner before interviewing them about the stress they had encountered the day before. The researchers then asked the ladies about the stress they had experienced. After the participants had finished their meals, the researchers checked their blood sugar, cholesterol, insulin, and cortisol levels, as well as their metabolic rates (the rate at which they burnt calories and fat), and evaluated their metabolic rates.

The findings of the study showed that women who reported experiencing one or more sources of stress in the preceding 24 hours burnt 104 less calories on average than women who did not report experiencing any sources of stress.

This might cause a weight increase of 11 pounds in the span of a single year. Women who were under a lot of stress also had higher insulin levels, which is a hormone that has a role in the accumulation of fat.

Poor Health Behaviors that are Caused by Stress

High levels of stress are experienced by those living in contemporary civilizations. Throughout the years, many different definitions for the concept of stress have been utilized. When trying to describe stress, one of the most important ideas to keep in mind is homeostasis, which refers to the intricate and ever-changing equilibrium that plays a significant role in the preservation of life.

When seen from this angle, stress may be understood as a state of danger or perceived threat to homeostasis, which the body responds to by activating a complex network of behavioral and physiological reactions to adjust to the new environment. The stress system, which is localized in both the central nervous system and in peripheral organs, is responsible for regulating the response that occurs in response to stress.

Because an increase in cortisol is one of the most prominent effects of stress, high levels of cortisol in the saliva and blood are generally regarded as the most reliable biological indicators of stress.

It has been demonstrated that the stress that individuals experience may cause physical, behavioral, and psychological problems. Some examples of this include headaches, constipation, smoking, alcohol misuse, poor food, sleep disruptions, and obesity.

People exhibit a behavioral shift toward a more westernized dietary pattern when they are under stress. This includes emotional overeating, excessive consumption of high-fat, high-salt, and high-sugar meals, and decreased intake of fruits and vegetables.

In addition to the changes in hormones that are caused by stress, it is also possible for stress to motivate you to participate in harmful activities that may lead to weight gain. These behaviors include the following.

Emotional eating: Not only may increased levels of cortisol make you want unhealthy food, but extra nervous energy can frequently encourage you to eat more than you would typically consume in response to stressful situations.

You could discover that eating or reaching for a second serving gives you some brief respite from your stress, but that doing so makes it more difficult for you to maintain your weight healthily.

Eating "accessible" or fast food: When we are under pressure and not making plans, we tend to eat the first thing that we see and/or what is readily available and accessible, which isn't always the healthiest option. When we don't plan, we tend to eat what is readily available and accessible, which isn't always the healthiest option. It's also possible that you'll be more inclined to drive through a fast food restaurant rather than spend the time and mental energy required to prepare a well-rounded, nutritious dinner in your own home.

Less physical activity: With all the pressures placed on your schedule, physical activity may be one of the things that fall to the bottom of your list of priorities. If so, you're not alone. There may not be a lot of opportunities for physical exercise if you have a lengthy commute and spend a lot of time sitting at your job.

Skipping meals: When you are juggling a dozen activities at once, having a nutritious meal might come down on the list of priorities. However, skipping meals can have negative effects on your health. You may find yourself missing breakfast because you're already running late or skipping lunch. After all, there are simply too many things on your to-do list. Both of these scenarios are understandable.

Less sleep: When worried, many individuals report having problems falling asleep or staying asleep. And studies have shown a correlation between not getting enough sleep and a slower metabolism. Having a lack of control and contributing to bad eating habits may also result from being overtired.

CHAPTER SEVEN

HOW TO ESCAPE THE NEVER-ENDIND CIRCLE OF STRESS AND OVEREATING

It's easy to neglect good activities like eating well and working exercise regularly when you're under a lot of pressure, like

when you're stressed out. Keeping a regular schedule and/or routine may help turn these healthy actions into habits and in preventing weight fluctuations that are caused by stress. The following is a list of some of the ways that you may interrupt the cycle of stress and weight gain for yourself:

Make working out a top priority. Getting regular exercise is essential to lowering stress levels and maintaining a healthy weight. Because it can help you address both problems at the same time, it is necessary for preventing weight gain that is caused by stress. Include some kind of consistent physical activity in your daily routine. This may be going for a stroll during your lunch break or heading to the gym after work.

Consume comfort foods that are better for you.

Carbohydrates and fats are not required to make you feel better at all. One of the few studies that have been conducted to test the effectiveness of comfort foods in improving mood discovered that eating relatively healthier comfort foods, such as air-popped popcorn, is just as likely to boost a negative mood as eating "unhealthy" foods. If you keep these kinds of foods stocked in your pantry, it will be much simpler for you to reach for a more nutritious option whenever you find yourself under a lot of pressure.

Eat with awareness and presence of mind. It's possible that eliminating distractions and concentrating solely on what you're putting in your mouth can help you feel less stressed, lose weight, and keep it off. According to the findings of one study, overweight women who participated in mindfulness-based stress and nutrition training were better able to control their emotional eating and had lower overall stress levels, both of which contributed to a gradual loss of abdominal fat throughout the study. Try eating your next meal without being distracted by your phone or the television the next time you sit down to eat.

Keep a record of the meals you eat. If you pay attention to your eating patterns, it will be easier for you to acquire control over the amount of food that you consume. Those who maintained a food diary had a greater chance of successfully managing their weight than those who did not keep a food journal, according to a review of research published in 2011 that investigated the connection between self-monitoring and weight reduction.

If you are more attentive to what you put in your mouth, you may be able to change your eating habits. This is true whether you use an app to monitor your food intake or you write everything down in a food diary.

Drink more water. It's simple to get thirst and hunger mixed up in your head.

However, conflating these two desires might cause you to consume more calories than your body requires, which can ultimately result in weight gain. After you have corrected any slight dehydration, it is considerably simpler to recognize the sensation of hunger.

If it's just been a couple of hours since your last meal but you're already feeling hungry, the best thing to do is start by sipping some water. If you still feel hungry after eating, you should have a snack.

Grab some protein

Protein is more likely to deliver the relief from stress that you are seeking for, even though tension may cause you to grab the next sweet or salty food. Tryptophan is an amino acid that is naturally found in foods including salmon, turkey, nuts, seeds, and cheese. Tryptophan is known to promote feelings of relaxation and overall well-being in humans. If you don't have time to make a complete meal, one of these scrumptious recipes for protein shakes will help you get more protein into your diet in a hurry.

Please inhale and exhale fully.

Taking a few slow, deep breaths may be all that's needed to bring your stress level under control. When you breathe in a leisurely and methodical manner, oxygen is drawn into your lungs.

This alleviates the nervous sensations that sometimes accompany being out of breath and, in the process, may calm down a heart that is beating too quickly. Researchers at the University of the Basque Country showed that deep breathing exercises helped lower cortisol levels in both male and female research participants. This finding suggests that deep breathing exercises may also assist you in reducing your body fat percentage.

Get Some Sleep

When it comes to relieving stress, sleep is almost incomparable to anything else. A good night's sleep may help your body fight off sickness, lessen physical discomfort, and eliminate the continual stress that is a part of your everyday life.

If you get enough sleep, these benefits can all be yours. Researchers from the University of Chicago and the Free University of Brussels discovered that even just one night of reduced sleep can increase cortisol levels the following day. This indicates that there is no better time than the present to begin enhancing your physical and mental health with some restful, in-depth sleep.

Although you may not be able to make your work simpler or add more hours to your day, there are still many things you can do to control your stress level and live a healthy life. You can get started on the road to a more relaxed you by making sure you get enough rest, that you engage in some regular exercise, and that you include the 50 Best Detox glasses of water for Fat Burning and Weight Loss into your usual routine.

Strategies for relieving stress should be included in everyday living. Whether you find peace in practicing yoga or reading a good book, consider incorporating basic stress relievers like taking a deep breath, listening to music, or going for a walk into your daily routine. These things may help you feel better quickly. Your cortisol levels may go down, which can help you keep a better handle on your weight management efforts.

www.ingramcontent.com/pod-product-compliance
Lightning Source LLC
Chambersburg PA
CBHW071946120726
48001CB00005B/2062